FRUCTOSE

MALABSORPTION

DEALING

WITH IT

MY WAY

LARGE PRINT

JOAN MAGUIRE

Copyright Page

New: Fructose Malabsorption Dealing With It My Way
Large Print

Author: Joan Maguire

National Library of Australia Cataloguing-in-Publication
– Publication entry

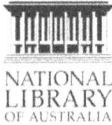

A catalogue record for this book is available from the National Library of Australia

Published with the assistance of CreateSpace and Draft2Digital is available through www.helpfuldietaryrecipes.com

Large Print version created on 7th February 2018©
ISBN: 9780648220619 (large print)

This short story book was created and written
By Joan Maguire on18th July 2017©
ISBN: 9780994543172

E-book written August 2017© and is available through the providers on www.songtitlebookss.com
EISBN: 978099454389

DEDICATION

I would like to dedicate this book and say
to thank you to my Earth Angel David
and his friends, who inspire and motivate
me to achieve things that I never dreamt,
were possible.

You have been my saviours many times
when I have wanted to give up on life

INTRODUCTION

This book is about my journey through the ups and downs of living with a virtually unknown medical condition known as Fructose Malabsorption. I know that there will be some people who will give me heaps of stick for writing it as they will say that it is not necessary for me to state what FM has done to me and what it is still doing to me. I am ready for your backlashing.

It's true, I don't need to write it down; however, it is necessary because other people can relate to what I am writing and because of this, they know that they are not alone and there is someone out there who cares. I will be straight forward in what I have to say and some of the things will not be very nice to read; however, it has to be mentioned and it will be the truth.

They say that Fructose Malabsorption is a complicated medical condition, and it is.

There are so many pieces to it that are only being discovered now and most times there are other medical conditions that people like me have to deal with as well. In this book I will give you the information that I have gathered for myself from many, many internet sites and it's a pity that a few of the really good ones are not on the net anymore. I will try to explain the different parts of Fructose Malabsorption, or as I sometimes call it FM, and some of the other medical conditions that can also be attached.

I am not qualified in anything so please don't think that I have every answer and that all the information is the gospel truth; in fact, a lot of the information on the different web sites can be very conflicting and only give the information that is required by their site.

I will not be talking about my past in any sordid details nor will I talk about my family. I will only mention my medical helpers, doctors and specialists using different initials or letters from my own name (Joan Patricia Maguire). I am a person who believes in strict confidentiality and most of my life is just that; confidential.

I hope that my story will help other people to understand what it is like to have a little known medical condition with very little help at hand. . It is a personal ordeal for each one of us and no-one can do anything about how we feel or cope with it.

ACKNOWLEDGEMENTS

I would like to thank my immediate family for their positive support when times for me were tough, even though they didn't know what I was going through at times.

I would like to thank the many, many people on the numerous web sites that have given me most of the information that I required at the time and still use often. I am not able to even name you all without writing another book.

I would like to thank the few close friends who have just sat and listened to me when I needed to talk; again they didn't really know what I was going through at the time.

I would also like to thank everyone else who has helped me bring this book to life and to you, I hope that it will be a learning experience for you and that you may be able to help yourself or someone else with some of the information that this book contains.

People, who know me, know that I am a Bon Jovi freak and I would like to say a special thank you to them, for their songs have meanings behind the lyrics that have pulled me through many bad times and make me feel good and more positive the more I listen to them.

I would like to thank all the other people, who shall remain nameless, you know who you are, for being there for me and going through the good and bad times that I have had without judgement.

OTHER BOOKS IN THE COOKBOOK SERIES

Helpful Dietary Recipes For Most
Intolerance

Helpful Dietary Recipes For Most
Intolerance
International Cuisine

Helpful Dietary Recipes For Most
Intolerance
Condiments

CONTENTS

THE EARLY YEARS

In the introduction I stated that Fructose Malabsorption is a complicated medical condition. Most people would know of Irritable Bowel Syndrome which is one of the earlier diagnoses for FM. There is a lot that I can say but I'm not going to as you will get the main gist from the story without a lot of repeats.

I was diagnosed with Irritable Bowel Syndrome way back in 1971 and was told then that it was brought on by stress and there was nothing that could be done for it.

As I sit here and write this, I am reflecting back to my past and remembering some of the little things that my mother had told me about when I was young.

My mother had told me that I was a very "windy" baby and she used to give me orange juice to help with my constipation, but it never did anything but make me worse.

This may have been the beginning of my issue and nobody knew of FM back in 1951 in England.

I was the second child born and I had an older brother. As the years went on I had two other brothers and then two sisters and none of them that I know of, had the issues that I have.

Dad had an allotment where he grew some of our vegetables, so we were all raised on a healthy diet. Mum also baked healthy snacks and cakes for us.

In 1957 our family came to Australia and we settled in Adelaide, South Australia where my father's parents and brothers lived. I don't really remember that much because I was still rather young but many photos from those years showed that I had a bit of a "pot belly" but none of my brothers or sisters had one.

I used to be known as "Fatty Patty" because my middle name is Patricia or Joanie and I used to become angry over it, so much that I used to hate my middle name and sometimes shorten my first name to Jo. I used to always keep to myself because of it.

Other girls my age wouldn't have much to do with me because I was "too fat" to fit in with their groups.

I was tested for Myopia (short sightedness) at the age of nine and had to wear glasses and these also were another form of name calling for me and another reason why I was not accepted by the other girls. I was "short and dorky", not tall and slim like them.

I was not the bright spark at school like my eldest brother was, so my schooling only lasted until I turned 16 years old when my mother took me out of school and sent me to work in a job that she had arranged for me but it didn't last long.

I tried to get into the Airforce but my height, weight and my eyesight let me down.

The recruitment officer stated that they could pass me by measuring me with my shoes on, they could get my weight down through the basic training but it was my eyes that was the issue. I had to see for a certain distance without wearing my glasses which I couldn't do.

My height stayed the same, my eyes stayed the same but my weight went up as I became bigger around the middle. I had trouble finding clothes to fit me so I started making my own and wearing the styles that I liked. Usually the clothes were not fitted ones and although they were loose on me, they were not baggy.

The style of fashion in the 70s and 80s helped a bit as there were many of them.

I had one friend from high school and we used to go out on weekends until her family moved interstate and I lost track of her.

I got into a small group of people and slowly I became an item with one of the guys.

He taught me to surf and how to pull out diffs and panel beat but it ended because his mother said that her son should find someone who was a lot prettier and slimmer than what I was.

I had a couple of other boyfriends but they didn't last long because someone would always make fun of them being with me, especially if I had had a drink and I started bloating.

The alcohol would give me wind/gas and I couldn't get rid of it so I began to look like I was pregnant. That look and all the torment that I went through in my past left me hating my body and myself no matter how hard I tried to change it.

Then one afternoon someone who knew me a bit introduced me to my now ex-husband.

MARRIED LIFE WITH FM

I bought a beautiful wedding dress but as the wedding drew nearer; my mother had to alter it because I began bloating more often, I kept getting bigger. Mind you, it would come and go and on my wedding day, my stomach had bloated in a way that I looked like I was in the early stages of pregnancy but my mother was able to fix my dress to hide it. I know she wasn't happy about the way I looked but she never said anything that day.

Not long after I was married, I fell pregnant with my beautiful eldest daughter, so I had an excuse for being "fat". This time people used to say that if I fell over, I would just lay there and rock back and forth. Another comment that hurt; however, I never showed my feelings because it always led to more nasty comments.

Two years after my first daughter was born, we found out that she had a serious medical condition and would need surgery. I was pregnant with my amazing second daughter and this news didn't help my medical condition at all.

With a new baby, a daughter who had just had major surgery I became most unwell and went to my doctor who informed me that I had Irritable Bowel Syndrome brought on by the stress I was going through and there wasn't anything they or I could do about it except to stop stressing. They also stated that I had a mental health issue (anxiety) and put me on anti-depression drugs.

Our diet had always been good and there was little that I had to do to change my eldest daughter's diet after her operation.

Two years later my wonderful son was born and a few years later things started to go wrong in my marriage. My husband found someone younger and slimmer than me and left to live with her, leaving me to raise my children. He would come back and we would move to another state to start a new life.

I will only say that this went on for thirty years but my self-confidence was gone, I hated myself completely and my so called IBS got worse. I only wore clothes that were size 20 or bigger.

Now, I stated earlier that I was short; I am 152cm tall or just a fraction over 5 feet so being the size I was didn't look good at all.

I was accused of being obese, lazy and a hypochondriac but I wasn't any of them.

I would go to the doctors often because of my bloating issue and all they wanted to do was to give me more drugs and suggested that I should find a counsellor.

My children had grown and left home and I got a divorce and sought help wherever I could find it. I also took up dancing 50s & 60s rock and roll and I enjoyed it very much.

It was a good form of exercise for me and a very good stress release. I had a dance partner but that was it; the past reared its ugly head again; I was good to dance with but the so called "package" was not good enough to be seen out with. I was too short and too fat. Bloated meant fat.

I decided to go back to study and get myself a career so I enrolled in a TAFE course to do Community Service.

Two years later, I left with four diplomas and three certificate fours in several branches of Community Service and Community Housing.

During two of my diploma courses I learnt about what drugs can do to your mental health and how to control and keep most mental health issue at bay. I was also very fortunate to have a very good doctor who would work with me and we would often exchange information and learn from each other.

I went to see my doctor, who I will call Dr. J, one day and it just so happen to be a really bad day for me and the bloating.

He couldn't believe that I could be so big that I had trouble breathing, let alone walking so he sent me for a blood test.

The results came back stating there was something wrong with my glucose so I had to have another test done where I had to blow up a helium balloon with a straw. The results came back stating that I was a Type 2 Diabetic. (FM was not known of at that time and the tests are the same)

Dr. J knew that my diet was based around me cooking and eating fresh vegetables and I ate very little junk food. I never ate fruit, drank alcohol, fizzy drinks or fruit juice because of the wind/gas effect that they would have on me. I did enjoy my tea and coffee though.

I am also a smoker so I tried some of the quit smoking products. One worked for a little while. However, my bloating became so severe that Dr. J arranged for me to have an Endoscopy done to find out what was wrong.

Two years after I was diagnosed as a Type 2 Diabetic I went in to have my Endoscopy done. Before I was wheeled in to the theatre, the surgeon (Dr. M) came out and asked me some questions; like my name, age and why I was there.

When I told him about my bloating issue he stated that it sounded like I have FM and have most probably had it since I was a baby but not born with it.

He also stated that it had only been discovered about eight to ten years ago and there weren't that many doctors who knew about it and there was some information on it but not much.

There wasn't really any specific tests that can be done to prove it so it would be all trial and error on my part.

Was this the reason I had been suffering all my life?

The following day I started my research on FM and cut all the vegetables out of my diet. I was fine eating meat and dairy. Unfortunately I was no longer able to enjoy my cups of coffee during the day and my tea at night because they both had Polyols in them. If I drank any sort of tea at night I would be awake around four in the morning with pains in my stomach that were like being in labour with my three grown children at the same time. The pain would not go until I passed the wind/gas.

When my stomach is so bad, I can't do anything. I get frustrated, go into a downward slide quickly into depression and I just want to give up on life.

It can take me anywhere between one week to a month to pull myself back into a sort of normal life. (More on that later)

I know that there are some people out there nodding their heads yes because they go through it as well. FM does control your life until you learn how to deal with it to suit your own needs. It does cause mental health issues due to the fact that eating out is very hard because you have to be very careful with what you put in your mouth and people won't invite you to join them because of it.

I went out to dinner with my daughters back in February 2017 and we went to a place where I knew I could eat certain foods like a chicken schnitzel; the only thing is the place now adds onion powder to the breadcrumbs and that alone gave me issue starting twenty minutes after I had finished eating and for the following three weeks.

There wasn't anything mentioned even after I had spoken to them about my FM. They didn't really listen to me and I was thought of as being fussy and they thought that I wouldn't even notice.

Yes, I have been to and spoken to many dieticians and other nutritionists who all think they know best about your body and they don't appreciate you saying otherwise.

I do have to mention this so please don't get me wrong because this happened to me. I went to see the dietician at the same hospital where I had my Endoscopy and she and I had a few words concerning the FODMAP diet. I told her that I had tried it before several times and my body couldn't handle it.

I have never seen anyone go into a tantrum so quickly because she knew what was best for me so to stop the tantrum I said I would try it again.

Thirteen days later I was back at my doctors with bloating, walking and breathing issues and he nearly had a fit when he saw me and I told him what had happened.

He gave me a good telling off and took me straight off the diet because it was killing me due to the wind/gas build up was squashing my lungs and my heart.

He sent me straight back to the dietician to let her see what she had done to me. The dieticians comment was "Well we had to try didn't we". There wasn't any apology from her.

I have tried seeing other dieticians for help and one teaching place actually asked me not to come back because I was too complicated and they couldn't help me and didn't want to know.

THE REASONS FM IS COMPLICATE

Don't forget that this is the research that I have found out to help me with my issue and it may not be correct and it may be conflicting to what you know. My main issue with FM is the Polyols; the sugar alcohols that not many health practioners from all areas know about or know little about.

I will also be putting in some information that I have taken from the net and if I can cite the web site then I will. Other information may be from my files or from web sites that are no longer available or just snippets from different web sites. Also the information may have come from one particular web site but it can also be found on other ones.

Please don't bite my head off if you think that I have used your information for my educational book and haven't acknowledged you but your site may not have been the one that I took it from.

All sites on these issues are helpful to me and other people; however, I may just be bringing it all together so I thank you for your long, hard and frustrating work.

Fructose Malabsorption is made up in a few parts. First there is Fructose which is the natural sugar in just about everything. Then there are Fructans which is mainly wheat products and is in some form in fruit and vegetables. Then there is the Polyols or sugar alcohol that is in everything. It is the natural sugar that God gave to each plant as a food source to help it grow. Then there is the Galactans which are also wind/gas causing parts in most foods.

A BRIEF SUMMARY ON FRUCTOSE MALABSORPTION

This information was taken from: http://www.marksdailyapple.com/fodmaps/#ixzz4Cqm7oyio
"You could be having a fairly routine conversation about health and nutrition where everything discussed is familiar.

You hear things like "carbs" and "medium chain triglycerides" and "fructose" and "macros" and "gluten" and "PUFAs," thinking nothing of it. Like I said, routine. Then someone mentions FODMAPs. Huh? What the heck is that?

Quite possibly one of the strangest, seemingly contrived acronyms in existence, FODMAPs represents a collection of foods to which a surprisingly large number of people are highly sensitive. To them, paying attention to the FODMAPs in their diets is very real and very serious if they hope to avoid debilitating, embarrassing, and painful digestive issues.

To begin, what exactly are FODMAPs?

As I said, it's an acronym:

F is for Fermentable – Fermentable carbohydrates are carbohydrates that are fermented by bacteria instead of broken down by our digestive enzymes. In most people, some fermentable carbohydrates are healthy sources of food for the (helpful) bacteria that ferment them; these can include the prebiotics I've championed in the past and can actually improve digestive and overall health. In people with FODMAPs intolerance, certain carbohydrates can become too fermentable, resulting in gas, bloating, pain, and poor digestion, as well as proliferation of unwanted pathogenic bacteria.

O is for Oligosaccharides – Oligosaccharides are short-chain carbohydrates, including fructans (fructooligosaccharides, or FOS, and inulin) and galactans (raffinose and stachyose). Fructans are chains of fructose with a glucose molecule at the end; galactans are chains of galactose with a fructose molecule.

D is for Disaccharides – These are pairs of sugar molecules, with the most problematic being the milk sugar lactose (a galactose molecule with a glucose molecule).

M is for Monosaccharides – This describes a single sugar molecule. Free fructose is the monosaccharide to watch out for with FODMAPs intolerance.

A is for And – Every list needs a good conjunction.

P is for Polyols – Polyols include sugar alcohols like xylitol, sorbitol, or maltitol. For an idea as to their effects, type one of them into Google and note the autofill choice (hint: it's usually "diarrhea" or "constipation" or "gas").

Since large amounts of polyols rarely occur in nature, lots of people have trouble with them.

The reality, of course, is that digestive difficulties are widespread, particularly in the industrialized world. If it's not constipation, it is diarrhea, or bloating, or gas, or hemorrhoids, or IBS, or all of the above. These complaints are sadly very common (even more common than the stats would suggest, since many people are too embarrassed to admit they have an issue).

For many of these people, FODMAPs may be exacerbating their symptoms.

Normal carbohydrate digestion takes place in the small intestine, where polysaccharides are broken up into glucose, fructose, and galactose and transporters like GLUT2 and GLUT5 absorb them for the body to use as nutrients. Sometimes those sugar molecules make it past the small intestine into the large intestine where colonic bacteria – the gut flora we (sorta) know and love – gobbles it up via fermentation, potentially causing gas and painful bloating.

The presence of too many sugars in the colon can also cause an influx of fluid, which could lead to diarrhea. Constipation is another common symptom, though it's not clear exactly how FODMAPs cause it. And some polysaccharides, like the oligosaccharides, make it through to the colonic bacteria as a rule because they resist digestion in everyone (in healthy people, these have a useful prebiotic effect).

You might be thinking, "Cool, so I can just avoid those weird sounding sugars and be fine, right?" Probably not. FODMAPs are very prevalent in the food supply. Even if you avoid free fructose, don't drink milk, and ditch processed food containing sugar alcohols, you'll still run into them in many fruits and vegetables.

FODMAP-containing vegetables include:
Asparagus (fructose, fructans), artichoke (fructose), beets (fructans), broccoli (fructans), Brussels sprouts (fructans), butternut squash (fructans), cabbage (fructans), celery (polyols), cauliflower (polyols), eggplant, fennel (fructans), garlic (fructans), leek (fructans), mushroom (polyols), okra (fructans), onion (fructans), shallots (fructans), sweet corn (fructose), radicchio (fructans), sweet potato (polyol)

FODMAP-containing fruits:
Apples (fructose, polyol), apricots
(polyol), avocados (polyol), blackberries
(polyol), cherries (fructose, polyol), plums
(polyol), pluots (polyol), lychees (polyol),
nectarines (polyol), peaches (polyol),
pears (fructose, polyol), persimmons
(polyol), grapes (fructose), mango
(fructose), watermelon (polyol, fructose),
dried fruit (fructose), juice (fructose)

Plus sweeteners like honey, agave nectar,
maltitol, sorbitol, mannitol, and xylitol.
And any dairy that contains significant
amounts of lactose, like milk or soft
cheeses. Depending on your sensitivity,
cream or butter can even do the trick.

So it covers quite a few otherwise healthy
Primal foods (and some non-Primal ones,
like wheat and rye and the
aforementioned refined sweeteners).

Let me reiterate before I go on, because
I don't want to scare everyone away from
berries and broccoli: not everyone has
problems with FODMAPs.

Most people probably don't. If you're eating all that stuff without issue, continue doing so and consider this post merely an academic curiosity.

Who might benefit from limiting FODMAPs?

Anyone with small intestinal bacterial overgrowth (SIBO)

Normally, the small intestine has relatively low numbers of gut flora residents. In SIBO, it's got tons that aren't supposed to be there. They interfere with nutrient absorption, digestion, and just generally muck everything up. SIBO has been shown to correlate quite strongly with lactase deficiency. Without enough lactase, you won't be able to digest lactose (one of the premier FODMAPs) and your colonic bacteria will have to do the job. Another, earlier study found that patients with SIBO also show malabsorption of fructose and sorbitol in addition to lactose; all three are FODMAPs.

Anyone with IBS

Low-FODMAP diets beat the pants off conventional dietary advice for people with IBS. One study found that while healthy subjects had increased flatulence on a high-FODMAP diet, subjects with IBS had increased flatulence in addition to lethargy and adverse GI symptoms. This could indicate that both groups were feeding FODMAPs to their gut bugs (which produce the flatulence through fermentation), but only the IBS patients had enough pathogenic gut flora to produce adverse symptoms.

Anyone suffering from chronic stress

Stress is a well-known disruptor of digestive function as anyone who's gotten queasy, lost their appetite, or had explosive diarrhea before the big interview could tell you. There's evidence that stress might be causing FODMAP-intolerance, too. First, stress inhibits the action of GLUT2, a transporter responsible for the small intestinal absorption of glucose, fructose, and galactose in the gut. If you're unable to adequately absorb the sugar molecules in the small intestine, they end up making it to your large intestine for fermentation by colonic bacteria. Second, stress has an immediate impact on the composition and function of your gut flora, rendering your populations less diverse and allowing certain pathogenic species to overpopulate.

Anyone with otherwise unexplained digestive problems
Maybe you haven't had a diagnosis. Maybe you just don't feel right after eating almost anything. Maybe you're chronically constipated (or the opposite). Trying a low-FODMAP diet can help you narrow your focus and start to identify some culprits.

If you decide to embark on a low-FODMAP diet, consider keeping a diet journal to log your food and track your reactions to individual FODMAPs.

Some people might really react poorly to fructose while having no issues with lactose. Point being: different FODMAPs affect different people differently. You can tolerate some and not others.

Dosage matters, too. A gram of inulin might be fine, while five grams could cause distress.

Individual tolerance must be determined by, well, seeing what and how much you tolerate.

If you're interested in healing your gut, whether from SIBO or IBS or anything else that might be predisposing you to FODMAP intolerance, well-established protocol like GAPS (Gut and Psychology Syndrome) diet or SCD (specific carbohydrate diet) may help and are worth looking into.

If you have no digestive issues, I would caution against trying a low-FODMAP diet "just because". You'll be missing out on some very nutritious, important foods, probably unnecessarily, while adding a bunch of unnecessary stress to your eating. FODMAP-related digestive issues are very noticeable. You'll know it if you have it".

Some people can be born with Hereditary Fructose Malabsorption or get it when they are babies. The surgeon who did my Endoscopy thinks that's when I may have got it.

Another snippet about Fructose Malabsorption that we need to remember comes from http://www.strandsofmylife.com/8-symptoms-fodmap-intolerance-explained/

"All fruits and vegetables contain fructose and many contain fructans and polyols, which can cause us folk problems.

Some are lower in these substances than others and so can be tolerated in small helpings. Your digestive system rules your life.

Of course, this rules your life.

I have always wondered what it would be like to not have to constantly think about this issue and how it would impact on each of my decisions in life. I know now because I have it under control – finally. I seldom worry about toilets any longer but must always be aware of what goes into my mouth. If I suffer or not is now up to me. Not to fate".

WHAT ARE FRUCTANS AND GALACTO-OLIGOSACCHARIDES?

This information was taken from: http://fodmapfriendly.com/what-are-fodmaps/what-are-fructans-and-galacto-oligosaccharides/

Fructans are fructose polymers and are the naturally occurring storage carbohydrates of a variety of vegetables, including onions and garlic, fruits and cereals.

Additional sources of fructans are inulin or Fructo-oligosaccharides (FOS). Inulin and FOS are increasingly being added to foods for their known prebiotic effects.

The human small intestine does not produce enzymes capable of hydrolyzing these fructose-fructose bonds and as such fructans cannot be absorbed across the small intestine. They are then delivered into the large bowel, where they can be readily fermented by colonic bacteria. Fructans alone can induce abdominal symptoms and can also exaggerate those associated with fructose malabsorption or lactose intolerance.

Hence, fructans are often limited in any dietary modification for patients with fructose malabsorption and IBS.

Like fructans, galacto-oligosaccharides or chains of galactose molecules are also malabsorbed in the small intestine. Individuals do not produce enzymes that hydrolyze galactose-galactose bonds and they too are readily fermented by bacteria in the large bowel. Significant dietary sources of galactans (raffinose and stacchyose) include legumes such as lentils, chickpeas and red kidney beans.

Vegetarians often consume large amounts of galactans due to increased consumption of legumes as they often provide an important source of protein in a vegetarian diet.

A little bit of information on Galactans: "Galactooligosaccharides (GOS) are short chains of galactose molecules that can cause symptoms due to fermentation. It should be noted that the GOS are generally found in legumes and seaweed and many foods have not been characterized regarding their GOS content".

Sugar Alcohols: Everything You Need to Know By Mark Sisson http://www.marksdailyapple.com/ sugar-alcohols/

I've been on a bit of an alternative sweetener kick these past few weeks, for good reason: people want and need to know about this stuff. While a purist shudders at the prospect of any non- or hypo-caloric sugar substitute gracing his or her tongue, I'm a realist. People are going to partake and it's important to understand what's entering your body and what, if any, effects it will have.

Whether it's diet soda, artificial sweeteners, stevia, or the mysterious sugar alcohols, people want the sweet without worrying about a big physiological effect – an insulin surge, a blood glucose dip, even a migraine. So I've been covering the various types and have tried to be comprehensive about it. As a whole, it all seems fairly safe. Alternative sweeteners might mess with some folks' adherence to a low-sugar diet, and they might induce or fortify cravings, but the research doesn't suggest that they're going to give you cancer or diabetes. The potentially negative effects are all fairly subjective, so it's safe to play around with them and determine their role in your life based on how they affect your appetite, state-of-mind, and any other subjective health markers.

One remains, however. I have yet to cover sugar alcohols. I was surprised, actually, having gone through my archives and finding nothing. Sugar alcohols are pretty prominent in the low-carb world – all those sugar-free desserts and chocolates and protein bars geared toward Atkins types tend to use sugar alcohols – so I had better get to it, huh?

What Are Sugar Alcohols?
A sugar alcohol, also known as a polyol, is an interesting type of carbohydrate. Its structure is kind of a hybrid between a sugar molecule and an alcohol molecule (hence the name "sugar alcohol") and, for the most part, our bodies do a poor job of digesting and breaking down sugar alcohol in the small bowel. It's also sweet to the tongue and resistant to fermentation by oral bacteria, meaning sugar-free gum manufacturers employ it judiciously to sweeten their products without causing cavities. Our colonic bacteria, however, can and do ferment the stuff.

For that reason, it's a kind of prebiotic that, as Kurt Harris points out, can stimulate diarrhea and exacerbate existing irritable bowel syndrome-related symptoms. Common side effects of sugar alcohol consumption (or over-consumption) include bloating, gas, and abdominal pain.

Sugar alcohols are not quite non-caloric, but all contribute fewer calories than sucrose, and their effects on insulin and blood sugar (if any) are pretty minimal.

Sugar alcohols pop up in nature, in fruits like apples and pears, but any commercial product that contains them must list the specific alcohols in the ingredients. If they aren't counted toward the official carb count, they must be listed separately in the nutritional information. Let's look at some of the popular ones you'll be encountering:

Xylitol – Glycemic Index of 13
Xylitol is one of the more popular sugar alcohols. It tastes remarkably like

sucrose, has about half the calories, and is 1.6 times as sweet, with little effect on blood glucose and none on insulin levels.

You can find xylitol in certain berries, corn husks, mushroom fibers, and oats; most commercial xylitol comes from hardwood and corn. Xylitol has a cooling effect on the mouth and is actively protective against dental caries (as opposed to merely being neutral or non-contributive, like the other sugar alcohols), making it the favorite choice of sugar-free chewing gum makers.

There appear to be some interesting health benefits to xylitol, too, beyond the well-established preventive actions against dental plaque and cavities. Xylitol shows promise as a bone remineralization agent, positively affecting both tooth enamel and bone mineral density (albeit, thus far, in rats). I count at least ten studies showing xylitol's promise in the treatment or prevention of osteoporosis. Just don't feed it to your dog. Also, it may exacerbate intestinal distress or cause diarrhea, so exercise caution (and linger near a toilet if you're unsure of its effect on you).

Sorbitol – Glycemic Index of 9
Sorbitol is found primarily in stone fruits, and manufacturers use it in diet sodas, sugar-free ice creams and desserts, as well as mints, cough syrups, and gum. It's about half as sweet as sucrose, with 2.6 calories per gram (compared to sucrose's 4 calories per gram, of course). Being a polyol, it has the potential to cause great gastrointestinal distress, especially in patients with IBS. This is compounded by its relative lack of sweetness when compared to other polyols, like xylitol; people are more likely to consume greater amounts of sorbitol to attain the desired level of sweetness and companies are more likely to use more of it.

There don't appear to be any proactive beneficial effects with sorbitol. It doesn't affect insulin or blood glucose, which could be good for diabetics, but there's nothing like xylitol's promise.

Erythritol – Glycemic Index of 0
Erythritol is almost non-caloric (0.2 calories per gram) and about 60-70% as sweet as sugar. It's the only sugar alcohol that doesn't appear to cause gastrointestinal distress (because the body absorbs it rather than let it pass to the colon for fermentation), it doesn't affect blood sugar or insulin, and it cannot be fermented by dental bacteria (and it exhibits some of xylitol's inhibitory effect on carie-causing oral bacteria, though not all of it).

For the most part, erythritol seems pretty safe, and it's rumored to taste very similar to sugar. Overconsumption – taking in more than your body can absorb – can result in bloating and gastrointestinal distress, but it takes a lot.

Maltitol – Glycemic Index of 36
Maltitol is very similar to actual sugar in terms of mouth feel, taste, and even

cooking performance (except for browning, which it cannot do). It's 90% as sweet with half the calories, so manufacturers love using copious amounts of maltitol in sugar-free desserts and other products.

That's all well and good while you're eating the stuff, but what about half an hour later once all that sugar alcohol has finally reached your colon and the bacteria has started feasting and fermenting?

Bloating, diarrhea, abdominal pain.

It's right there in the name, isn't it? Mal.

There are others, but those are the big ones. Overall, the literature shows that sugar alcohols are fairly neutral as far as blood glucose and insulin effects go. Some people may see spikes, as I've seen reports on blogs and in comment boards to that effect, but most people won't. They can hit your gut pretty hard and cause problems there, especially if you've got a pre-existing condition, but healthy people with healthy digestion (which isn't as widespread as most people think, of course) should be okay with some here and there. Xylitol in particular seems promising, and I'll keep my eye out for more information on that as it emerges.

If you're doing fine without sweeteners (non-caloric, hypo-caloric, artificial, natural, whatever), keep it up.

Don't go looking for an excuse to introduce sugar substitutes.

But if your desire for something, anything sweet is derailing your attempts at a healthy diet, sugar alcohols may be worth experimenting with. Give it a shot if you're gonna and let me know how it goes.

What have your experiences been with sugar alcohols? They get a bad rap from being used in so many processed "low-carb" treats, but have they helped or hindered your path to health?"

Here's a list of some popular sugar alcohols so you can identify them when you look at a nutrition label:
Erythritol
Maltitol
Hydrogenated starch hydrolysates
Isomalt
Lactitol
Mannitol
Sorbitol
Xylitol
Methanol or aspartame

Aspartame/methanol (unknown source maybe from my files)

Aspartame is most often labelled as containing phenylalanine.
Aspartame is made up of aspartic acid and phenylalanine. The latter has been synthetically altered to carry a methyl group, which is responsible for aspartame's sweet taste. The phenylalanine methyl bond, called methyl ester, allows the methyl group on the phenylalanine to easily break off and form methanol.

In fruits and vegetables, methanol is bonded to a fiber called pectin that allows it to be safely passed through your digestive tract. However, in aspartame, methanol is not bonded into anything that can help eliminate it from your body.

Once inside your body, the methanol is converted by alcohol dehydrogenase (ADH) enzyme into formaldehyde, which can wreak havoc on your DNA and sensitive proteins. All animals, except humans, possess the ability to break down methanol into formic acid.

Methanol, also known as wood alcohol, is found in antifreeze and rocket fuel, among many other applications.

Methanol's effect on the body is similar in some ways to that of ethanol (the alcohol found in wine and beer), but unlike ethanol, the body deals with methanol by transforming it into waste products that include formaldehyde, a carcinogen that morticians use as embalming fluid.

If aspartame delivers methanol to your bloodstream, it would seem like a no-brainer to avoid the sweetener at all costs, but there's a confounding factor: methanol is also found in all sorts of harmless foods, especially fruits and vegetables, in quantities comparable to foods that contain aspartame. In fact, aspartame-flavored soda contains less than half the methanol found in the same volume of many fruit juices.

This is where the dialogue gets contentious. To some researchers, it's clear that methanol is harmless in the small quantities derived from aspartame-containing foods.

However, a study conducted in 2005 by the European Ramazzini Foundation, which tracked the health of aspartame-fed rats for their entire natural lives, linked aspartame consumption with an increased lifetime cancer risk.

Some researchers, as well as the U.S. Food and Drug Administration, found fault with the study's methods, while other scientists rushed to defend it, saying that at the very least, aspartame requires continued examination.

At the heart of the debate is the fact that in rats, as in humans, a large percentage of individuals will succumb to cancer in very old age.

It's difficult for scientists to say whether cancer in a very old rat was caused by lifetime ingestion of a substance such as aspartame, or whether the cancer would have occurred naturally.

As I mentioned in the Introduction, there are other medical conditions that people may also have with their FM issue and some that I was unaware of until I wrote my second cookbook.

Here are just three more little known medical conditions that other people with FM have to deal with;

OXALATES AND SALICYLATES: http://www.pkdiet.com/pdf/oxalate%20lists.pdf

"Some folks are particularly bothered by oxalates and salicylates, which are plant chemicals and yet, if they were to ask their physicians about them, would find no answers concerning them.

Oxalates are chemicals in plants (and some animal foods) that bind with minerals in the body, such as magnesium, potassium, calcium, and sodium, creating oxalate salts. Most of these salts are soluble and pass quickly out of the body. However, oxalates that bind with Calcium are practically insoluble and these crystals solidify in the kidneys (kidney stones) or the urinary tract, causing pain and irritation. Oxalates, as far as I know, are not used in products but as flavourings for recipes. One spice is Cinnamon that is a very high oxalate spice with over 38 mg of oxalate for just one teaspoon. Choose instead cinnamon oil or cinnamon extract.

Cinnamon oil is available from various outlets that sell culinary oils. You can get cinnamon extract in the supplement section of your grocery or health food store – generally, it is sold in capsules. When cooking with it, you simply open the capsules and put the powdered extract into your dish. Substitute about the equivalent amount of dry extract for ground cinnamon. (Not sure about here in Australia).

Salicylates are natural chemicals found in plants that protect the plant from being eaten by insects or attacked by disease. Although poisonous, salicylates are usually tolerated when ingested in small amounts, but when ingested too frequently, they can cause a wide range of symptoms. Salicylates are found to a higher degree in unripe food. This poses problems for Americans, as our food is often picked way too early.

Salicylates are used to make prepared foods, hygiene (toothpaste, lotion, soap, etc.), cosmetic, and drug (Aspirin and others) products, which we are also using more and more of".

For confidentiality reasons, I have edited the next section for this book.

FOOD INTOLERANCE NETWORK FACTSHEET

https://fedup.com.au/factsheets/additive-and-natural-chemical-factsheets/amines

AMINES

Introduction

All foods are made up of hundreds of naturally occurring compounds that can have varying effects on us, depending on how much we eat and how sensitive we are.

Biogenic amines are formed by the breakdown of proteins in foods. They can affect mental functioning, blood pressure, body temperature, and other bodily processes. Some hormones, such as adrenaline (epinephrine) are compounds containing an amine.

There are many different amines, including:
- tyramine (e.g. in cheese)
- histamine (e.g. in wine)
- phenylethylamine (e.g. in chocolate)
- agmatine, putrescine, cadaverine, spermidine (e.g. in decomposing fish)
- tryptamine
- adrenaline (ephinephrine)
- serotonin
- dopamine

Biogenic amines are normally quickly broken down in the body with the help of enzymes such as MAO (monoamine oxidase-A) which render them harmless. Missing, sluggish or blocked enzymes can lead to a build up of amines in the body.

The 'cheese effect'. In people who are taking certain drugs known as MAOIs (monoamine oxidase inhibitors), the enzyme is inhibited and a build up of tyramine can occur, leading to life-threatening high blood pressure as well as a range of symptoms including headaches, itchy skin rashes, heart palpitations and diarrhoea. A number of MAOI patients died from strokes or heart attacks before doctors realised that patients taking MAOIs needed to avoid foods high in tyramine.

This is called the 'cheese effect' because it was recognised in the 1960s by a British pharmacist who noticed that his wife developed a headache every time she ate cheese - high in tyramine - while taking MAOI antidepressants.

Lacking the enzyme. There is a rare condition in which people who are born without the MAOA gene lack the MAO enzyme.

Researchers have long known that this condition is associated with aggression in men.

Low activity enzyme. Much more common is a low activity variant of the gene known as MAOA-L, which seems to occur in about one third of the population. A study with nine uncontrollable children in 1985 found that on average there was five times more para-cresol in their faeces than for a control group. Para-cresol is a breakdown product of tyramine. Could it be that these children were failing to metabolise dietary tyramine due to a sluggish enzyme? We don't know because the study was never followed up, although the researchers commented that 'the results point to dietary involvement'.

In 2002, a study found that men with MAOA-L who had been badly treated as children were more likely to exhibit antisocial behaviour than those who had been well treated.

Amines and specific symptoms

Behaviour

Behavioural effects fit with what we see in the Food Intolerance Network. Children with oppositional defiance are the ones whose parents are often told 'he just needs a good smack'. But smacking has the opposite effect – if you smack these kids, when they are big enough they will hit you back. Or if they are scared of their parents, they will hit other people, and this is defined as conduct disorder. You have to treat these kids as if they are your friend – a calm approach – and avoid backing them into a corner at all times. It can be difficult to maintain a calm approach with someone who is extremely aggressive, and experts acknowledge that this approach has limited success. Network members find that it is easier to avoid the food chemicals that cause these effects.

Research suggests that about 70 per cent of children with behaviour problems are affected by salicylates, artificial colours and preservatives, compared to only about 40 per cent affected by amines. Many mothers have reported that their child becomes silly and hyperactive on salicylates whereas amines make them aggressive. In our experience, children who are expelled from day care centres due to aggressive behaviour are usually sensitive to amines as well as to other food chemicals.

Migraines, depression and other symptoms

Amines have been associated with migraines and headaches, as well as other symptoms of food intolerance, including irritable bowel symptoms, eczema and depression.

A possible link with schizophrenia

A biogenic amine called dimethyltriptamine (DMT for short) is the only known hallucinogenic compound naturally produced by the body. Normally it is metabolised by the monoamine oxidase enzyme before its effects can be noticed.

It is used in tribal and religious rites in South America by combining a naturally rich source of DMT with a natural MAO inhibitor while avoiding tyramine containing foods, usually through fasting. DMT is present in small amounts in a wide range of animal and plant foods and mushrooms. In the 1950s, researchers suggested that the schizoid symptoms of auditory or visual hallucinations could be due to an inborn deficit in the MAO enzyme, allowing small amounts of DMT from foods to build up in the body. This theory is once again becoming popular. It would account for why some failsafers have reported that schizoid symptoms improve on a low chemical elimination diet.

Amine levels in different foods

Fish, cheese, wine, some meats, some fruit such as bananas and avocados, some vegetables such as mushrooms, and fermented foods such as chocolate, sauerkraut and soy sauce are just some of the foods that have been listed as containing varying levels of amines, but basically any protein food can contain amines depending on the way it is handled.

The amine content of foods varies greatly due to differences in processing, age, ripeness, handling, storage, variety of grapes or other produce, cooking method and many other factors. An Australian analysis of the amine contents of fish-based oriental sauces found up to 6 times the legal limit of histamines in some of the samples. Freshness is a key factor for avoiding amines. The new method of meat distribution in our supermarkets is a problem for amine responders. All meat is now vacuum packed, repacked and sold as fresh which means it can be up to ten weeks old when you eat it.

Studies show that vacuum packing can inhibit the growth of bacteria but does nothing to retard the development of amines.

Many drugs can contain amines, including over the counter cold tablets, decongestants, nasal drops or sprays, some pain relievers, general and local anaesthetics and some antidepressants.

In 1996, researchers in a medical journal reported a more user-friendly MAOI diet based on laboratory analyses, claiming that many dietary restrictions were not necessary. Doctors on an internet forum were reluctant about advising patients to relax their diets. 'It is easy but is it safe?' asked one.

Another reported a patient whose diet infringement with a now supposedly safe food resulted in headaches, high blood pressure and seizures.

Experience suggests that people who are sensitive to amines need to know a lot of about the history and freshness of their foods and approach all possible amine-containing foods with caution. Lists of amine-containing foods (such as the one on the World Headache Alliance website) are not complete from our point of view. People with migraines who have avoided some amine-rich foods often say 'I tried avoiding foods and it didn't work'. This is because migraines can be provoked by many other amine-containing foods and/or other food chemicals such as additives, salicylates and glutamates.

AMINE INTOLERANCE OR ALLERGY: WHAT ARE THE SYMPTOMS?
http://whatcanieat.com.au/a/amines--salicylates/amine-intolerance-or-allergy-what--are-the-symptoms-

Let`s start by looking at what Amines are

Amines are naturally occurring chemicals found in many foods. They result from the breakdown of proteins or through the fermentation process, and are responsible for giving the food its flavour. The more intense the flavour, the higher the amine content, so the longer, say, a fruit ripens or a meat cures the more amines it will contain. The highest amounts can be found in aged cheeses, chocolate, wine, many alcoholic beverages, aged meats such as sausage or salami, canned or smoked fish, banana, avocado, and tomato. Amine content increases as certain fruits ripen and as meats and fish age, so those sensitive should only consume the freshest produce, meats and fish.

When you eat a food high in amines, the histamine it contains is metabolised by enzymes and bacteria to amines which are quickly absorbed in the gut and, in people who are sensitive, an allergy-type of response occurs.

The end result is widening of blood vessels, tissue inflammation and swelling just as our own natural histamine creates.

Amine Intolerance or Allergy: What are the Symptoms?

Symptoms of an amine allergy or amine intolerance usually depend on the amount of amine you eat you are likely to tolerate smaller amounts than larger amounts and occur when the enzymes responsible for breaking down histamine are saturated, or used up. The most common symptoms experienced by those sensitive to amines are recurrent eczema and hives, headaches or migraines, sinus trouble, mouth ulcers, fatigue (frequently feeling rundown and tired for no apparent reason), nausea, stomach pains, joint pain that is undiagnosed and digestive issues.

Children can become irritable, restless and exhibit symptoms related to ADHD.

Breast fed babies can exhibit colic, diaper rash, loose stools, and eczema through the milk if the mother is taking in excessive amounts of amines.

If you know that you have reactions to wines, aged cheeses or chocolate, there's a good chance you may be reacting to other foods high in amines. Take them out of your diet completely for a few weeks and see how you feel. If you do have sensitivity to amines, you'll want to limit the amount you eat every day, and determine what your own personal tolerance is to these highly reactive chemicals".

I know that there are a multitude of other well-known medical conditions and many more unknown medical conditions that require special diets; however, I am lucky in many ways that I only have FM to deal with along with the Diabetes, Irritable Bowel Syndrome and Depression.

If I keep my Fructose under control; then I can usually keep the other three conditions under control as well.

Again I state and please remember that I am not qualified in any field of medicine or nutrition and can only share my findings with you for many of the foods that I eat and these sites have similar information as other sites have.

Please listen to your own professional advisors and your own body and make sure that you seek the proper advice and not do a self-diagnosis because of the information that I have provided.

MY STORY CONTINUED

Now you know something about my issue, I will carry on with my story.

After a year of not having my beloved vegetables, I started craving them and my body was also telling me that it wanted them too so I started researching recipes for meals that I might be able to adapt for me to eat.

Again there were different sites that had recipes, mostly all American, but some of their ingredients were unavailable for me here in Australia and the substitutes were not suitable either due to the Polyols in them.

I made many phone calls and visits to dieticians who were not able to help me because they knew little about the Polyol side of FODMAPs. In fact; I taught some of them a little about them.

I still tried to eat some vegetables; however, I still ended up with the bad bloating and severe wind pains.

I found that I could eat just a little fruit if I cooked it with both Glucose Syrup and Dextrose Powder which is glucose in a powdered form.

I visited Dr. J for my regular check-up and we spoke about the bloating and pain issue again and he arranged for me to have a Colonoscopy done by Dr. M, the same doctor who did my Endoscopy, because he knew about FM. The results were that he couldn't find much wrong and I now have Diverticulitis which occurs when the bulging sacs that appear in the lining of your large intestine, or colon, get acutely infected or inflamed and pain on the lower left side of the abdomen.

Now to help with the Diverticulitis I have to drink plenty of water and eat fiber-rich foods like plenty of vegetables; especially the green ones. Oh great, how can I eat the vegetables to help with this new issue when the vegetables are one of the main reasons why I get the pain and wind/gas in the first place?

It was back to the drawing board and vegetable trying again. I tried each vegetable separately to find out which ones were not good.

I thought that I had some success with a couple of vegetables only to find that they were giving me issues in a severe way on the second or third try.

Now comes to the part where I am being honest and you won't like reading this.

I can't burp and passing wind/gas from the rear can sometimes be hard and when it does start coming it won't stop.

I am known to have my own "Farty Parties". The worst times are when I go shopping and right in the middle of my shop, I start breaking wind/gas while I'm walking so I have the embarrassment of not being able to control what is happening from my gut and having to get out of the shopping centre as quickly as possible and then having to catch two buses home.

Too much wind/gas in my stomach bloats me up that much that it has started to squash my lungs making it both difficult for me to breath and walk and gives me severe chest pains. I have even been rushed to the Emergency Department of two different hospitals because of the chest pains; however, once I get rid of the wind/gas I am alright. They thought that I was having a heart attack.

For me to get rid of the wind/gas from my system; I have to stick my finger down my throat and use it like a tongue depressor. This is extremely uncomfortable and dangerous due to the damage that I can do to my throat.

I have had to get up during the night to manually get rid of the wind/gas. Some weeks I have had to manually get rid of the wind/gas every day, or twice a day, for four or five days straight and that leaves me with a very sore throat and a couple of times I have scratched the back of my throat that bad that it has bled.

This also frustrates me and upsets me that much that I start going into depression. I know when I am going into a deep depression because I get Claustrophobic and all I want is a big long hug and I feel very unwell.

I try to stop this by taking myself on a two hour round trip on the Brisbane River or I jump on a couple of buses and head to the ocean for a while. I also have photos of my family around my living area so I can see them and I talk to my father and mother quite often. They are not the only photos that I have to look at and talk too; I have a particular male, who shall remain nameless, sitting on my table and stuck to the chair opposite me and gee do I give it to him sometimes or I should say a lot and all he does is sit there and smile at me.

Yes, he is someone who makes me feel good, lets me know that I am not alone in my place and he is someone who I can talk to in anyway I wish and I can have my silly fantasies and dreams.

In the end, I know where my feet are; planted on the ground, even though my head and mind are floating around in the stars.

These are safe coping measures for me as well as watching Bon Jovi concerts and listening to their music CDs.

I don't watch TV due to the ads and the negativity in different programs that are on plus I can't sit still even when I'm writing my books.

Some people think that I should get rid of my pictures; however, they don't realize the comfort and the positive mindset that they give me.

Without them I may have committed suicide a few years ago when the times for me were bad.

There are times when they are not that much better for me now; however, I'm alive and live day to day and do the best I can to keep myself busy and keep my mind concentrated on writing my books. (I'll tell you about them in a minute)

Many times I have started the day bloated and as the day went on, I lost the wind/gas and my clothes would have fallen off if my hips weren't there to hold them up. That is a good feeling and I haven't done anything different; it's my body doing it all by itself.

Also when I am in depression, I don't do anything; I mean nothing but play my Nintendo.

I have crossword games that are getting boring because they are so repetitive.

I had one game that I borrowed from my daughter and I used to enjoy playing it until I became obsessed with it and it used to infuriate me to the point where I would get very angry and I just wanted to throw it against the wall. I gave it back to my daughter and told her to never give it back to me. I don't want to eat, drink or even have a shower or get out of my nightie.

Claustrophobia usually starts setting in around these times; the walls start closing in around me making it harder for me to breathe. Even sitting outside doesn't help; however, I know that it will pass and I just have to work my way through it the best that I can. Going out would help but I can't be bothered. One side of my brain keeps giving me ideas to get myself moving but the other side says "That's what you think. Come back another time".

Other people like Dr. P (Dr. J retired) and my one close friend who I see regularly, think that I am eating well and I am very positive and doing really well; they don't know, but will now, that I don't eat. No food means less wind/gas and not having to rip my throat apart trying to get rid of it and I drink less water than I used too which is not good.

I have always had to hide my feeling so I am good in covering things up that I don't want people to see or know. I could be as low as I can get, yet I will still make people laugh and if my sense of humour is gone then run like hell away from me or you will cop it with both barrels.

Oh, I am surviving and I keep my Glucose levels fairly even but that is because I don't eat after seven in the evening but I do have a couple of small cake slices that are made with glucose after I have done my blood sugar reading before I go to bed.

Yes, I do get hungry to the point where I am shaky and feeling weak but I will have a drink of water and still not put food into my mouth.

I stated earlier in the book that I am a smoker and I know that I should give it up and believe me I have tried without success. Tobacco has methanol or aspartame in it so every time I go outside for a smoke, I give myself a dose of Polyols that I have issues with. I only have five smokes a day and that is too many.

STAYING SANE

For me to stay sane means that I have to keep myself busy; keep my mind occupied. Mind you it never stops thinking of new ideas or how to renew old ideas.

One of my main ways in keeping sane and making me want to live is spending time with my daughters over at my son's place just listening to the conversations that are going on and listening and watching my grandchildren playing and having fun. This is one time that I do eat because I enjoy the simply cooked meals and company but none of them know this until now.

I do have my Spiritual side that is very strong so that is another thing that keeps me going and sane and that is all I'm going to say on that subject. As Bon Jovi would say "Keep the Faith" and I do keep mine.

After leaving TAFE, I went and worked in a Community Housing Organization and in 2009 the organization closed its doors for good and I was unable to get another job.

In 2010 I was watching a Bon Jovi concert with a neighbour and I picked up the DVD cover and put the song titles into a sentence. My neighbour then got me to write the song titles into a short paragraph.

We both had a laugh and I thought that I would use all the song titles I had on every concert and DVD that I owned by Bon Jovi and write a small story and it didn't matter how many times the song title was repeated. I had found something new that I enjoyed doing that occupied my mind and time.

That story became the first of my thirteen published short story books. One of my daughters helped me financially and we found a publisher to help me publish seven of my book.

I was now an Indie author and was published without a big expensive book company backing me. My publisher made me a website but unfortunately the marketing side was difficult to do without spending heaps of money that I didn't have to get someone else to do it for me.

I found a Print on Demand publisher in America, CreateSpace, and uploaded all my books on their site for printing. I then found an eBook publisher, Draft2Digital and uploaded my books to them and they supply about eight eBook distributors like Apple and Kobo.

I then went back and changed all my print books into large print books for the visually impaired, uploaded them and they are all for sale. I do know that Amazon carry some of the books.

I learned how to make my own covers for the different books and I wrote, made my own covers and published six more books under the "Song Title Series" books.

Even though my thirteen books are still under that title, the website is no longer there but a new website "Song Title Books" now exists thanks to my brother.

Meanwhile my FM was still playing up and my body wanted the vegetables back. So it was back researching more information about Polyols and looking for recipes. Most of the good sites that I got my information from are now gone and most of the recipes are not really suitable for me so I started to copy and paste and adapt recipes that I could cook.

I came up with some interesting and flavoursome recipes but I ended up with the same issues, bloating and wind/gas and manually have to get rid of it which meant more sore throats. A couple of people became interested in the different recipes that I had made and asked if they could be adapted for Gluten Free and Lactose Free issues.

Cutting a long story short I was able to adapt them and then when I had finished, I had a very big cookbook written; 394 pages to be precise.

I was very proud of what I had achieved and the information that I was able to share. I emailed a few places to get permission to use some of their information in my book and when I received their permission, I uploaded my cookbook under the title of "Helpful Dietary Recipes For Most Intolerances" to both CreateSpace, my print place and Draft2Digital, my eBook distributor.

During all this work, I still tried to eat vegetables and found that I could eat potatoes without issue occasionally and I was also able to tolerate the Gourmet or exotic mushrooms. Enoki and oyster mushrooms are the best tolerated because they have little to no mannitol and xylitol in them; yes, those ugly Polyols again.

By this time I was getting mighty bored with the meat in my diet. How many ways can you cook chicken without getting sick of it? I started looking for different ways to cook it and get a different taste for it.

Dear old research came in again and my mind started working overtime giving me different ideas and I sent out ninety four emails to different cultural organizations that I used to deal with asking for some cultural recipes that they made but using ingredients that they purchased here in Brisbane.

Twenty two different cultures supplied me with quite a few recipes and after looking at them, I contacted them back and asked if I could use them in another cookbook.

That is how the "Helpful Dietary Recipes For Most Intolerances International Cuisine" was born. During the writing and research for this book, I became aware of two more intolerance, Oxalates and Salicylates, and decided to add them into the book.

The idea is to make other people aware of what is in all the foods we eat that people don't want you to know about plus it is a guide for people who have just been diagnosed with FM and the two other little known medical conditions; in fact, any medical condition that involves a diet change.

I struggled for help and information when I was first diagnosed with my medical condition and I assume that other people have had the same struggle when diagnosed with their medical conditions. I am only telling my story hoping that I may make it easier for someone else out there.

Again I state that I am not qualified in any medical profession of any type; I am just me on a journey looking for something to eat that I can tolerate.

My love of cooking and my imagination will not let me give up even though I still have my wind/gas issue that brings me down to very low levels and depression. I will not be beaten by FM or rather Polyols.

I would dearly love to get back to writing my Song Title Books again; however,

I haven't finished writing my next book "Condiments". Again this will be a book that has recipes that I am cooking and trying myself and it will have different ways to make homemade condiments that use the best ingredients that suit me and like the other books will have suggestions and some of the recipes will be left as is.

I have cooked so many different recipes that I can't eat; however, I have given the different foods to other people who have some of the issues and to a Community Organization that has a kitchen where people from different cultures come together.

I have my ingredients that I use and you have yours because you know what you can tolerate so this is where you can get new ideas for your meals. I have just had my half yearly check-ups and tests done and a couple of the results have come back better than what they were since the last lot of tests.

WHAT DO I EAT?

It is suspected that I have the Glut enzymes missing from my small intestines so therefore my body can't break down the foods I eat there. The food is broken down in the large intestine or colon and that is why I have the wind/gas issues and why I have to really watch what I eat and drink.

Not everybody has this issue but I do have it and I have to learn to work with it and live with it. I don't want it to run my life and continually send me into depression anymore. I've been in the depression era and worked my way out of it and off all the medication so I don't want to go back there again, I want to live and enjoy my life and have no more battles with my body and mind over what I want to eat or drink.

Well, obviously I don't have many vegetables except for the occasional potatoes, Shiitake, Enoki, Oyster and King Oyster mushrooms and on the very rare occasion I may try another vegetable just to see if it still does affect me.

I have found that I can still have the taste and colour of tomatoes; however, it is the skins that I actually dry, process down and add to my baking as I can tolerate them this way.

Most herbs are out; however, coriander is something that I can tolerate so I use that a lot. Again I usually dry it and add it to my baking.

I eat mostly lamb and chicken, a little pork and very little beef unless I mince it down. Bacon and ham are other meats that I can tolerate well. Fish is out because I have reactions to it like an allergy.

The occasion fruit like apples, cranberries and blueberries that are cooked in glucose syrup and dextrose powder are used in my baking.

I make breakfast slices made from oats, almond meal, rice flour, normal flour, cream, cinnamon and anything else that I have on hand. I change the ingredients to keep them interesting.

I like my eggs and hard cheese so they are in my diet a lot. I don't eat a lot of bread anymore or have cooked rice or pasta or Gluten Free products as they are all high in carbs which is not good for the Diabetes. Because I have a lot of protein, I am starting to get gallstones.

The green vegetables are important for your body and if you can't eat them, well, somethings got to give somewhere. I think gallstones or wind/gas and the gallstones win hands down due to what I will have to go through otherwise. This is what I have to think about and make a decision on everytime I want to put something in my mouth.

What will the consequences be and am I willing to take the chance? The answer is don't eat and no problems.

I am not Gluten Free or Lactose Intolerant; however, I don't mind Lactose Free cream cheese, liquid cream or milk for my baking.

The only lentils I have are yellow and green split peas that I make my own Pea and Ham soup with. Mind you I do have to soak the peas for at least twenty four hours using a lot of bicarb soda and changing the water often. It used to be a weekend job but now it is a three day job but it is worth it.

When I'm out and about, I find food that I can tolerate most times; like an egg and mayo sandwich. I say most times because here in Australia, companies tend to put garlic and onion in their mayo and call them spices. Garlic in mayo is really Aioli but you know how sneaky these big companies can get.

Garlic and onions are right on top of the no-go foods for me and just a little will give me very big issues that can last for days, even weeks.

I tend to use a lot of Rice Bran Oil as I don't like the taste of Olive Oil and I can't stand the smell of vegetable or canola oils anymore. Reports say that Rice Bran Oil is right on par with Olive Oil; maybe a fraction better with the vitamins.

I tolerate Nuttelex Original very well so I use that to spread on my crackers or toast with my vegemite but not very often and I tend to use it most in my baking. I can also tolerate one brand of Peanut Butter.

I also use a lot of rice malt syrup and dextrose powder because they are Fructose Free when I cook although I can have sugar if I want to.

I can tolerate one brand of coffee that I have in the mornings and a certain brand of iced coffee that I have a mug of in the afternoons if I am home. If I'm out and about, I tend to buy the iced coffee and drink that instead of eating. I drink water for the rest of the day. I have tried Milo and a homemade version of it but I still got the issues so I won't even think about having them again.

Through writing my cookbooks, I have come to know a lot about what is naturally found in foods that we eat and how they can affect you. If you don't have medical issues then you are able to get away with eating them and think nothing of it; however, if you had to stop eating them for some reason, then you would miss them and know what I am talking about.

Life can be very hard and trying for everyone; however, healthy people have no idea what it is like when your diet makes life harder for you and people no longer want to know you because they feel that they might catch what you have even though it is not contagious.

Yes, Fructose Malabsorption is a complicated medical condition that can leave you isolated, hating yourself and depressive and there is not a thing that you or I can do about it except to find our own ways of dealing with the issue and keeping ourselves positive and sane.

As I finish off this story I would like to let you know that it has been a hard, emotional ride for me as I have put in writing some of the things that happen to me that I would have preferred to keep secret. I am not looking for sympathy or anything like that. Don't waste your energy on feeling sorry for me for what I have been and are going through; put your energy to good use and keep yourself as healthy as you can be and help at least one other person along the way.

I would like to thank again all the people who have tirelessly put their time and effort into supplying the information that I have given.

Please check their sites out as they may have more information on it that you may be looking for.

Somewhere along the line I will start eating again; however, for now I will refrain from putting too much in my mouth if it is going to give me some relief from my issues and I will keep playing my Bon Jovi and talking to my family and "my man" as I call him. I will also be talking to the main man in my life and I will keep the faith that I have in him.

I will keep writing my books and keep hanging on to my dreams and my ultimate goal. I will stay positive and I will NOT let the Polyols win and get me down too often.

Everyone is entitled to get down in life; the important thing is not to stay down for too long.

Believe in yourself and you can get yourself up and about again and you will learn how to do it more often. I know it is easier said than done but you CAN do it if you put your mind to it and try.

MY FOOD CHART

As I have stated a lot in the previous pages that foods give me issues; this is part of the chart that I have made that shows what is in the foods we eat.

Now remember that my main issue is with Polyols; however, Fructose, Fructans and Galactans must also be taken into account as they usually go hand in hand and even in small amounts, together they can add up to big issues with me.

After the charts, I have placed a few interesting websites that talk about Methanol, Ethanol and Aspartame. Polyols usually end in ol, so anything that ends in ol is not a good option for me to have.

In my chart I have been able to identify some of the Polyols or Fructans; however, I am still trying to identify more and everyday some new information is found and I add it to the list.

Some sites will only say if they are Low FODMAP and to me it seems that they don't know what is in it. I call these sites copycat sites because what one site says is reflected on other sites because one person says so, it must be true. Sorry, but even Australian sites are like that and not up to date with information.

When I research information, I usually skip or just skim through the first page because I get more and better information on pages 2 and 3 that answer my question plus there is a certain University in America that is doing more work with the Polyol side of food. I know that researching takes a lot of money and time; however, for people like me who need certain information, these sites are virtually useless as they don't really cover Polyols.

I am going to use the following code system against ingredients as full charts for fruit, vegetables, herbs and spices would be very hard to read as some of them have all the following in them for example:

Mushrooms have HF (high Fructose), FOS (Fructans), PO (Polyol) (mannitol & xylitol) and GOS (Galactans) (raffinose)

Bananas have MF (medium Fructose), FOS (Fructans) (inulin), PO (Polyol) (sorbitol) and GOS (Galactans) (raffinose)

Fructose – F, Fructans – FOS, Polyols – PO, Galactans – GOS

Low – L, Medium – M, High – H, Very High – VH,

If one of the above is not listed, it will mean that the food item has either not been tested or it doesn't have it in it. There may be "EX" before the food item and that means that it is extremely high. MH means medium – high.

Acorn Squash	F, PO
Alfalfa Sprouts	HF, FOS
Almonds	F, FOS, PO (xylitol)
Aloe Vera Juice	PO

Amaranth (Gluten Free)	FOS
Apple Cider	F, PO (sorbitol)
Apple Cider Vinegar	F, PO (sorbitol)
Apple Juice	F, PO (sorbitol & methanol)
All Apples	F, FOS, PO (sorbitol), GOS (raffinose)
Apricots-Fresh	F, PO (sorbitol)
Asparagus	HF, FOS, PO (mannitol)
Aspartame (methanol)	PO (methanol)
Bananas	F, FOS (inulin), PO (sorbitol), GOS (raffinose)
Basil	F
Bean Sprouts	F, FOS
Beetroot	HF, FOS, PO (mannitol), GOS
Blackberries	F, PO (sorbitol & methanol)
Blueberries	F, PO (xylitol)
Borlotti beans	FOS, GOS (raffinose)

Broad / Fava Beans	F, FOS, PO, GOS
Broccoli	HF, FOS, PO (sorbitol), GOS (raffinose)
Brussel Sprouts	HF, HFOS, PO (sorbitol & methanol) GOS (raffinose)
Butter Beans	FOS, PO, GOS
Cabbage Green	HF, HFOS, PO (sorbitol), GOS
Cabbage, Red	HF, HFOS, PO (sorbitol), GOS
Cabbage - savoy	HF, HFOS, PO (sorbitol), GOS
Canned Fruits	HF, PO (aspartame)
Canned Vegetables	PO (aspartame)
Canola Oil	F, PO
Capsicum All	HF, FOS, PO (sorbitol)
Carrots All	HF, FOS, PO (sorbitol & methanol), GOS
Cashews	F, FOS, GOS

Cauliflower	F, FOS, PO (mannitol), GOS (raffinose)
Celeriac	F, FOS, PO (mannitol)
Celery	HF, FOS, PO (mannitol)
Chard	F, FOS, PO (sorbitol)
Cherries	F, PO (sorbitol)
Chick Peas	FOS, GOS
Chili Peppers powder/flakes /sauce	F, PO (mannitol)
Chinese Choy sum	FOS, PO, GOS
Chives	F, FOS, PO (mannitol), GOS (raffinose)
Chocolate / cacao powder	HF, FOS, PO, GOS
Choko	F, FOS, PO (mannitol)
Coconut	HF, FOS (inulin), PO (sorbitol), GOS

Coffee beans and instant	F, FOS, PO (mannitol), GOS
Corn	HF, FOS, PO (xylitol)
Cranberries	F, PO (mannitol)
Cucumbers	HF, FOS, PO (sorbitol)
Currants all	HF, PO (mannitol)
Curry powder	F
Dates	HF, PO
Dill	F
Eggplant	F, FOS, PO (xylitol)
Eggs	VLF
Endive	LF, FOS, PO (xylitol)
Fennel (not seeds)	LF, FOS, PO (mannitol)
Garbanzo Beans	FOS, GOS
Garlic	F, FOS, GOS
Ginger	F, FOS
Golden Syrup	F
Grapes all	F, PO (sorbitol)
Grape Juice all	F, PO (sorbitol & aspartame)
Green Beans	HF, FOS, PO (sorbitol)

Haricot Beans	FOS, PO, GOS
Honeydew melon	F, FOS, PO (sorbitol)
Kale	F, FOS, PO (sorbitol), GOS
Ketchup	HF, FOS, PO (methanol)
Kidney Beans	FOS, GOS
Kiwi fruit	F, PO (sorbitol)
Leek	F, FOS, PO (mannitol), GOS
Lemons	F, PO (sorbitol)
Lentils -Boiled	FOS, GOS
Lettuce	HF, FOS, PO (sorbitol)
Lima Beans	F, FOS, GOS
Limes	F, PO
Mandarin Oranges	F, PO (sorbitol)
Maple Syrup	F, PO
Mushrooms not exotic	HF, FOS, PO (mannitol & xylitol),GOS
Mustard seed spice	F, FOS, GOS

Nectarines	F, FOS, PO (sorbitol)
Olives	F, FOS, PO
Onions all	HF, HFOS, PO (mannitol), GOS
Orange Juice	HF, PO (sorbitol & aspartame)
Oranges	F, PO (sorbitol)
Oregano	F
Paprika	MF
Parsley	F, PO (mannitol)
Parsnips	F, LFOS, PO (methanol)
Passion Fruit	F, PO
Peaches	F, HFOS, PO (high sorbitol)
Pears	VHF, PO (sorbitol)
Peas	HF, HFOS, GOS
Peppers all	HF, FOS, PO (sorbitol), GOS
Pineapple	F, PO (sorbitol & mannitol)
Pineapple Juice	F, PO (mannitol & aspartame)
Pinto Beans	FOS, GOS
Plums	F, PO (high sorbitol)

Pomegranate	HF, MFOS, PO (sorbitol), GOS
Potatoes all	HF, FOS, PO, GOS
Pumpkin	M-HF, FOS, PO (mannitol)
Raisins	VHF, PO (sorbitol)
Raspberries	F, PO (xylitol)
Rice all	FOS
Rock melon	F, PO
Shallots (White part)	M-HF, HFOS, PO (mannitol)
Silverbeet	F, FOS, GOS
Snow peas	HF, HFOS, PO (mannitol), GOS
Spinach	HF, FOS, PO (sorbitol)
Strawberries	F, PO (xylitol)
Sugar snap peas	HF, HFOS, PO (mannitol), GOS
Sweet Potatoes	HF, FOS, PO (mannitol), GOS (raffinose)
Swede	FOS, PO
Tea all	PO (sorbitol)

Tomato juice, paste puree, Canned	HF, FOS, PO (mannitol & aspartame)
Tomatoes Sun Dried	F, FOS, PO (methanol)
Tomato soup	F, PO (mannitol & aspartame)
Tomatoes-Fresh	HF, FOS, PO (mannitol & aspartame)
Turmeric	LF
Turnip	MF, LFOS, PO (sorbitol)
Watermelon	F, FOS, PO (mannitol)
Worcestershire sauce	F
Zucchini	HF, FOS, PO (sorbitol)

I hope you can understand the coding in the chart because it was really the only way to put it without having a big mess that would have been harder to read due to the font size needed for this book.

Well as you can see, I don't really have much of a choice in what I eat. Some of the readings may be low in their category; however, put a few readings together and they become high and I am unable to tolerate them.

Most of the vegetables listed above is what my daily diet was based around for nearly my whole life, so getting FM and not being able to eat them anymore has been a great shock to my system and that is why I have been trying to put some of them back into my diet in one way or the other.

This is also why I have published my first two cookbooks and following them up with the "Condiments" cookbook so other people like me can have new choices and different ways to flavour and eat their food.

I hope that this book has enlightened you about Fructose Malabsorption and please remember that this is about me, how I deal with FM and why I can't eat the food that I should be eating **and** I am not qualified in anything to do with any part of the medical profession.

I have had to have a forced break during the completion of this book because through manually relieving my wind/gas about a fortnight ago, I seriously pulled muscles in my left side and rib cage. The pain became that bad that an ambulance was called. I was not able to do very much or wear underwear for nearly ten days. This was due to the fact that I ate a "safe" food; something that I had been able to tolerate many times before but now had onion and garlic in.

Please keep yourself as healthy as you can be and maybe help someone else along your journey in life. If they try to tell you about what is not working for them in their diet; don't laugh at them like people do to me because it only makes them feel worse.

I have only become aware of the following sites in the past day or two and

I found most parts of them interesting. I am not a rocket scientist so I didn't really understand the other parts. Please read them.

Websites
http://thetruthaboutstuff.com (and) whilesciencesleeps.com

http://observationhubie.blogspot.com.au/2006/05/methanol-talking-points.html

https://www.wellbeing.com.au/body/nutrition/aspartame-is-a-poison-not-a-sweetener.html

https://cot.food.gov.uk/sites/default/files/cot/cotstatementmethanol201102revjuly.pdf

www.ingramcontent.com/pod-product-compliance
Lightning Source LLC
Chambersburg PA
CBHW070526030426
42337CB00016B/2125